ISBN:
Hardback 978-1-922593-02-3
Digital   978-1-922593-03-0

BB & Tills Publishing

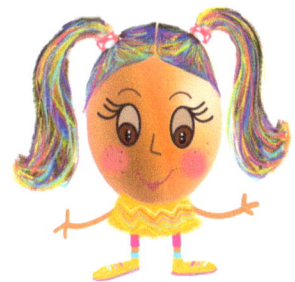

For Billie, Matilda, Amelia, Lucien, Ben, Daniel
and humans of all ages living with allergies.

Special thanks to Rosee Maxwell, Letizia Petti, Elizabeth Gilmore
and the countless others around the world who have
kindly gifted their time, support and feedback.

———

Proceeds donated to
Allergy Life Australia & Allergy Support Hub

———

This book contains stock photography, royalty free images
and the author's personal photographs.

Thanks to all the photographers!

©Peg the Egg was designed by Amy Marley.

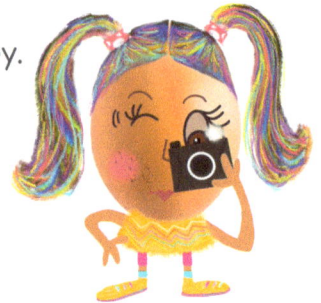

Preface

Peg the Egg is an introductory resource for kids of all ages to read with their parents, families, teachers, carers, specialists and whoever will read it with them!

Before reading this resource with a child, it is recommended you review the photos and text.

Some photos used may be disturbing.

Each of us are at different stages of the allergy journey and nobody processes the journey in exactly the same way.

You may feel certain parts are not yet appropriate. No right, no wrong — only what suits you and your family.

This resource doesn't have to be read all at once. Dip in and out of the information as needed.

As a parent new to the allergy journey, I found it challenging to manage risks day to day.

Reactions can be rare, so it isn't always easy to comprehend what is involved until the moment is lived.

My daughter was one when she had her first anaphylactic reaction to peanuts. We learned she was at risk of anaphylaxis to peanuts, tree nuts and eggs.

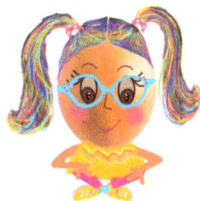

By the time she was 3 and off to kindergarten, she was still learning what nuts and eggs were and could barely say the word "anaphylaxis."

Our family's allergy journey expanded when my youngest had her first anaphylactic reaction to egg at the age of 4.

My intention has always been to empower them with information to self-advocate in a world filled with distractions.

The use of photos vs illustrations ensures there is no room for "make-believe".

Allergies are REAL.
Reactions are REAL.

While we can't allergy proof the world, using our voices and sharing information is a powerful way to expand the awareness of allergies.

Share your story.
It needs to be heard.

Please reach out to talk to someone if you are feeling excess fear or anxiety while managing allergies. There are psychologists, counsellors and support groups who specialise in navigating the allergy journey.

A list of resources is available at
https://amymarley.com/resources/

THIS BOOK SHOULD NOT BE RELIED
UPON AS AN ALTERNATIVE TO DOCTOR'S ADVICE

Each allergy case is different

Please see your doctor to confirm individual requirements

Peg the Egg

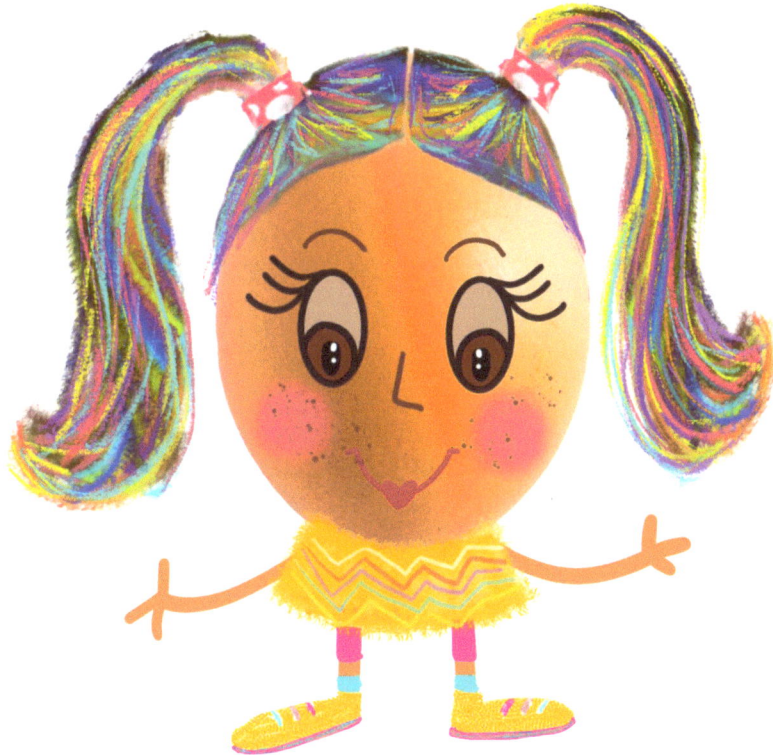

An Introductory Resource to Allergens, Allergies & Anaphylaxis

by Amy Marley

This is Peg. Peg's an egg.

Say hi, Peg.

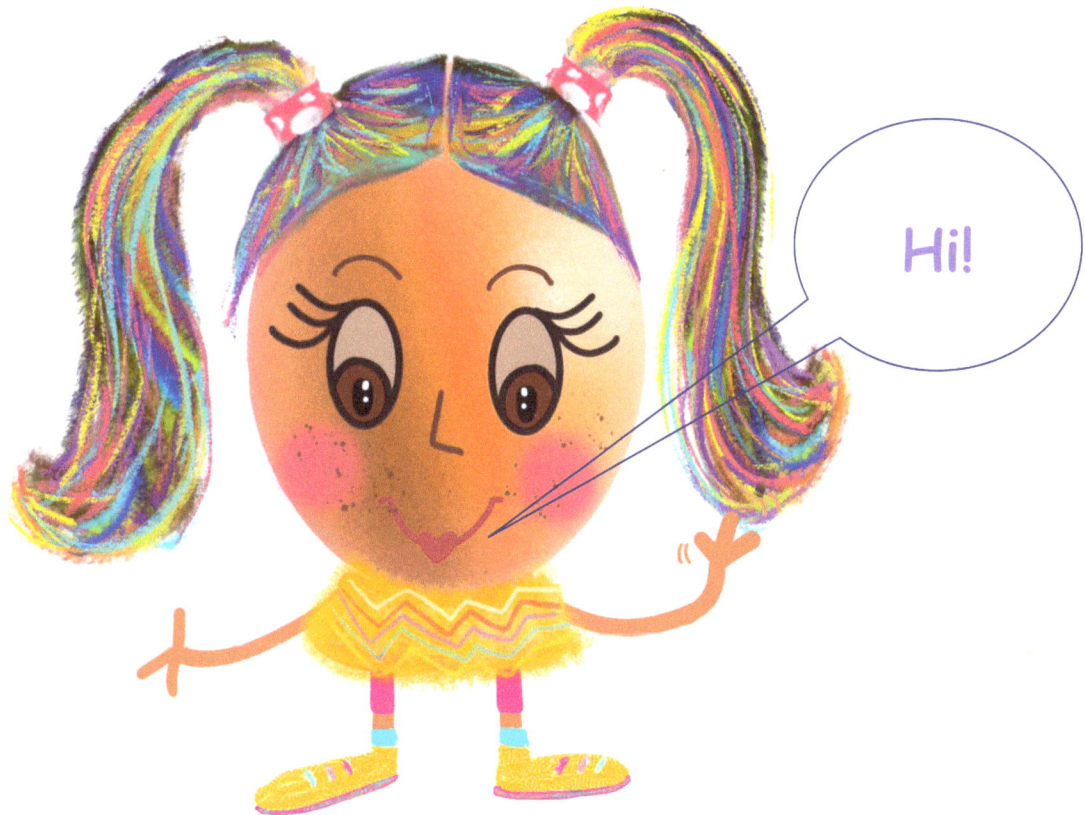

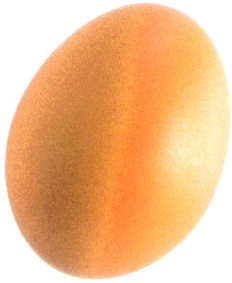

This is Peg in her shell

Peg cracked

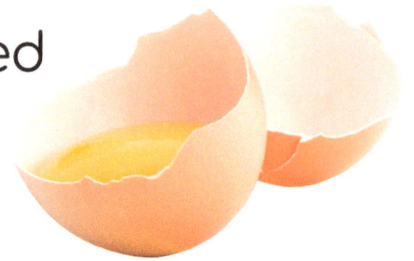

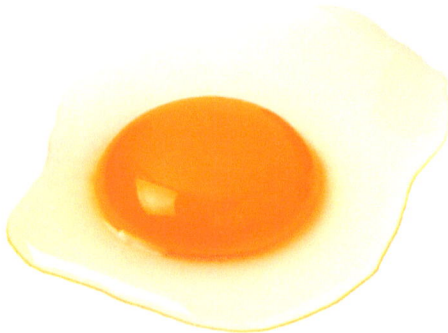

Peg raw

and Peg — *powdered!*

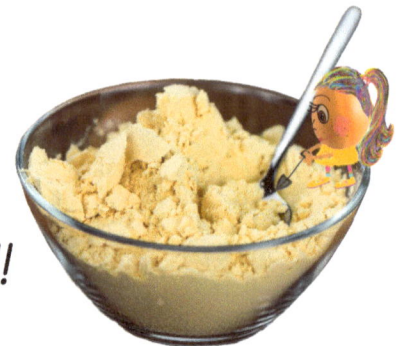

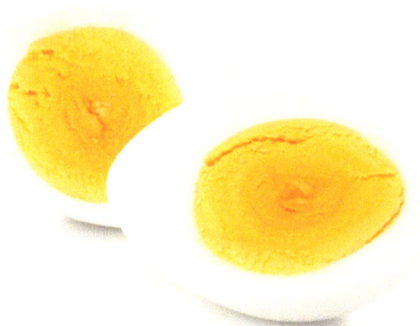

This is Peg boiled

Peg fried

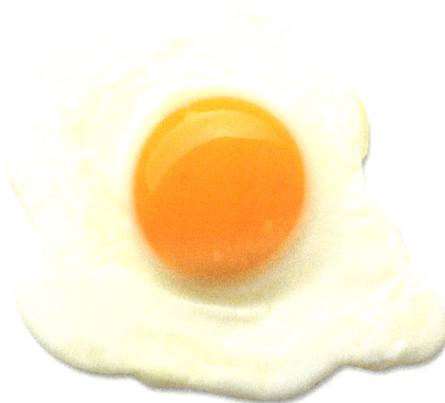

Peg poached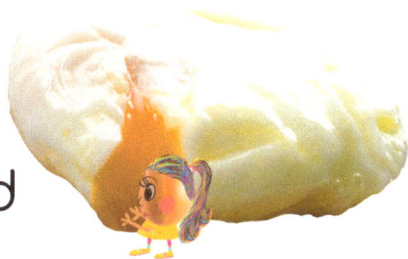

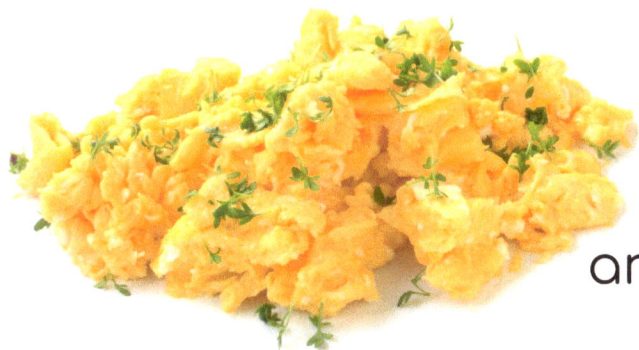

and Peg — *scrambled!*

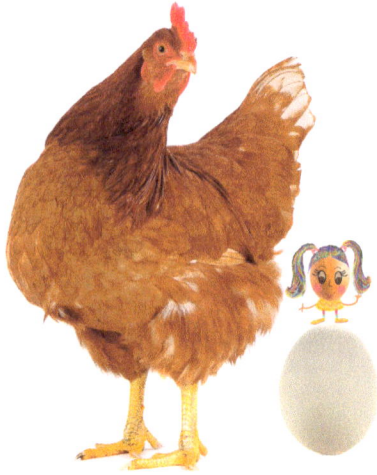

Peg was laid by a hen - the most common type of egg people eat.

Other types of eggs people eat are laid by

turkeys

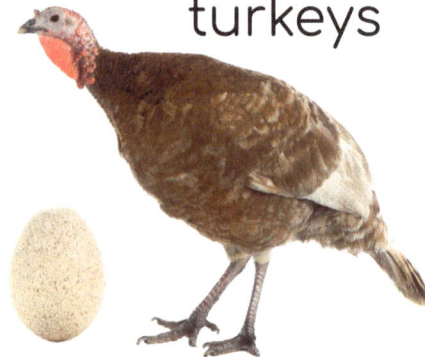

geese

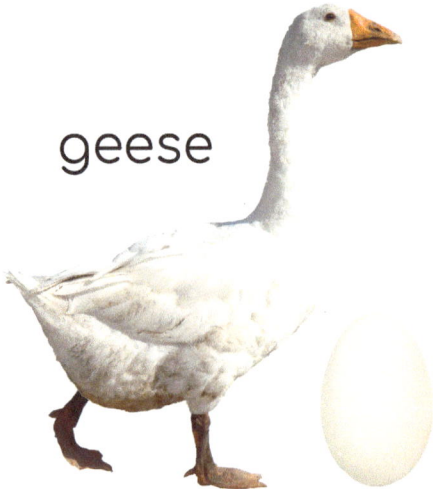

ducks

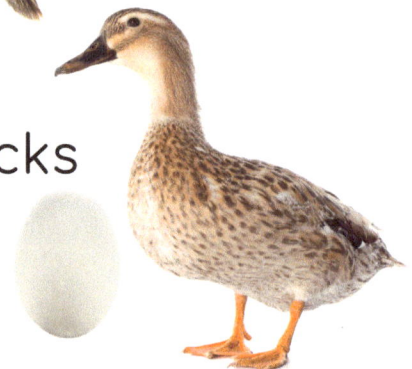

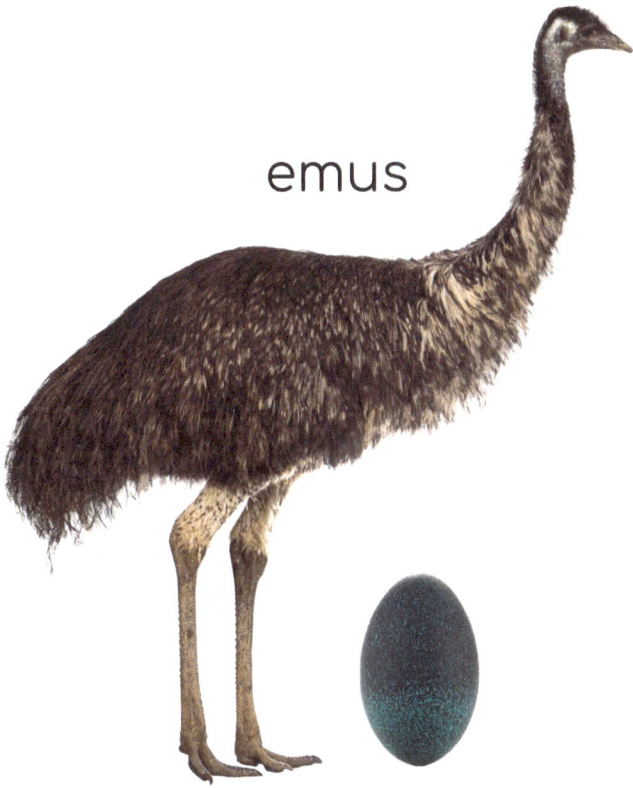

emus

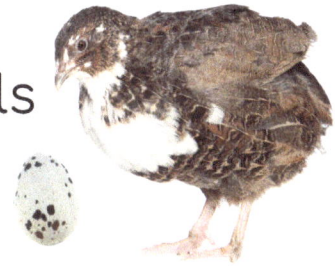

quails

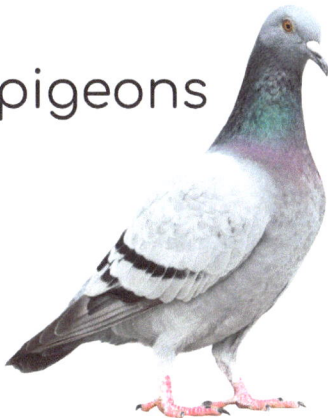

pigeons

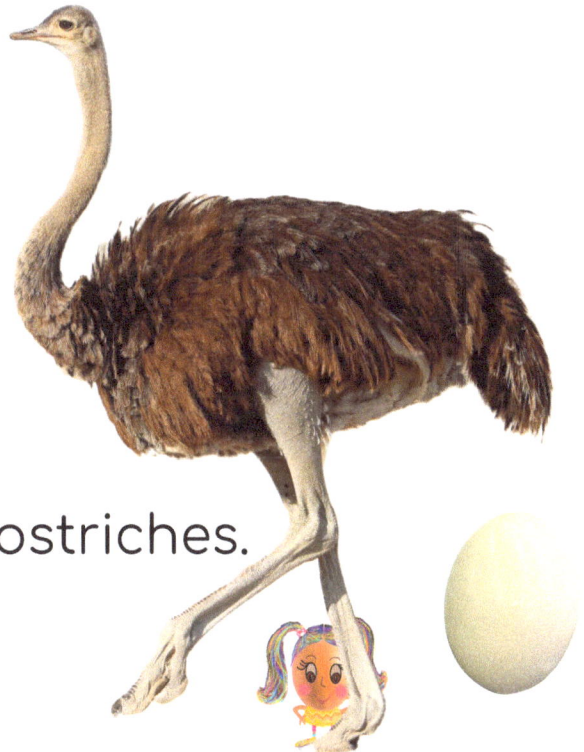

and ostriches.

Peg can trigger allergic reactions
in people who have allergies.

Let's find out more about
Peg and allergies.

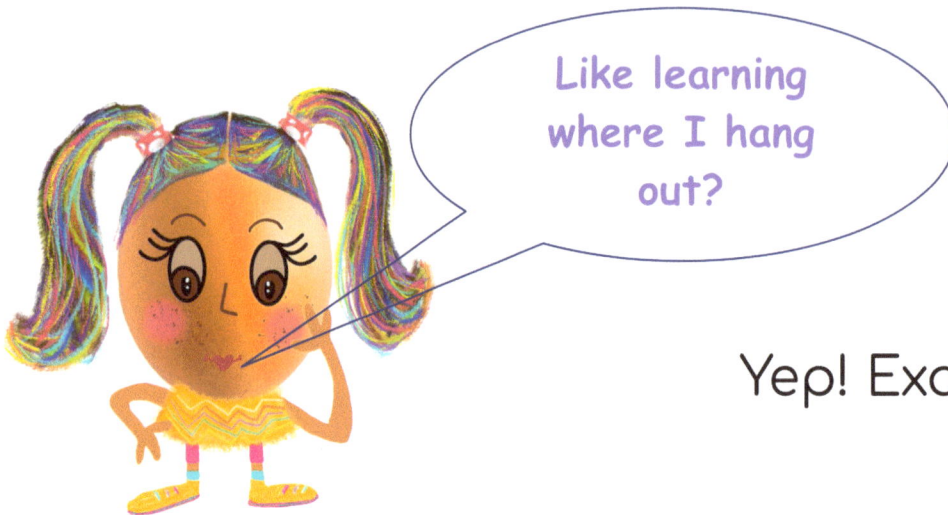

Like learning where I hang out?

Yep! Exactly, Peg.

Peg likes to hang out with other eggs in food like

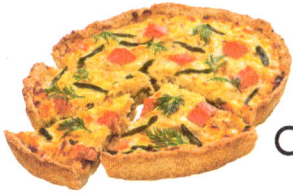

quiches, tarts

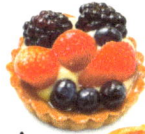

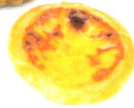

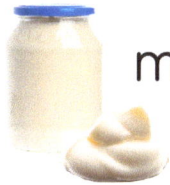

mayonnaise

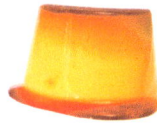

custard, curds and souffles

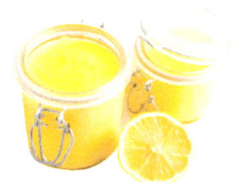

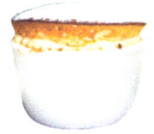

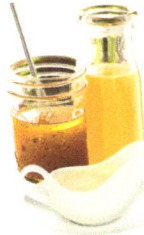

sauces and dressings

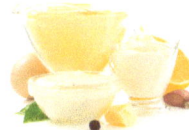

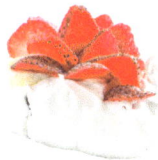

pavlova, macaroons and meringues.

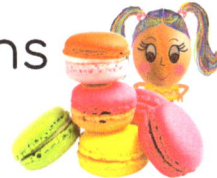

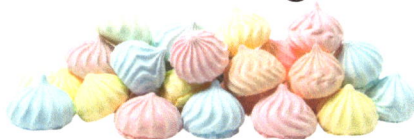

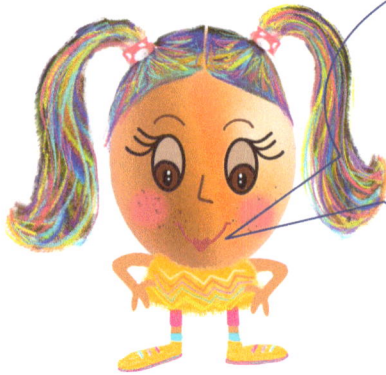

I can also be an ingredient in foods like...

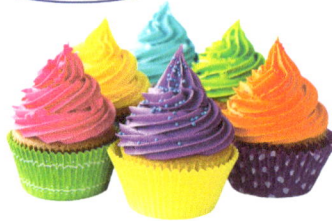

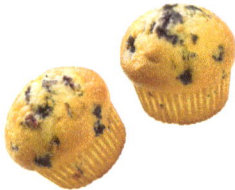

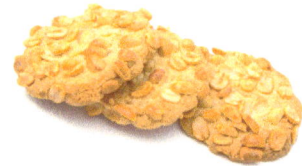

baked treats

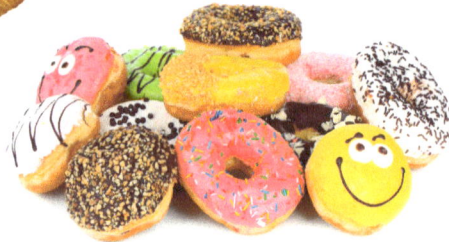

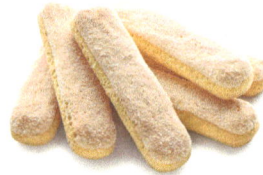

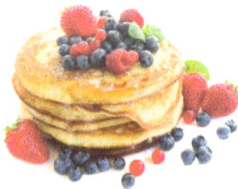

pancakes, waffles, pikelets, french toast

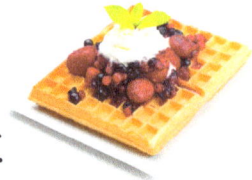

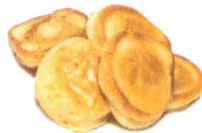

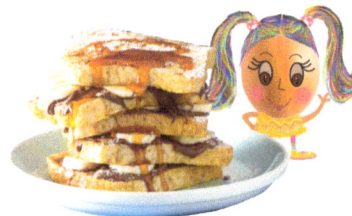

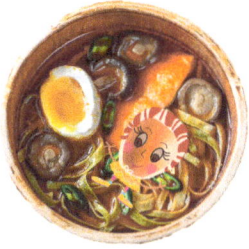

soups, stocks, salads

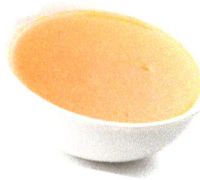

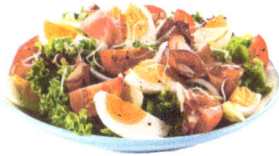

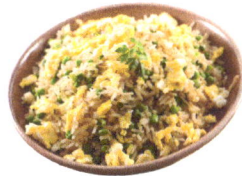

rice dishes

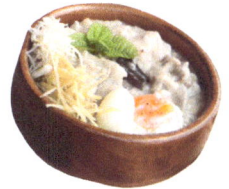

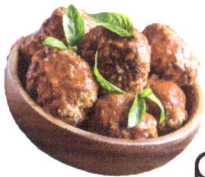

meatballs, pasta, noodles

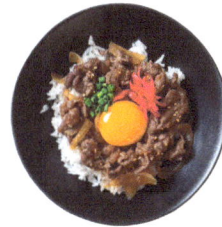

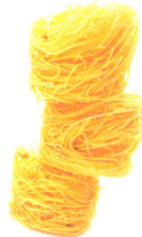

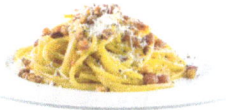

and fancy finger foods like dips, canapes and sushi.

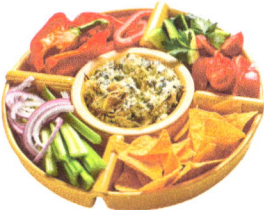

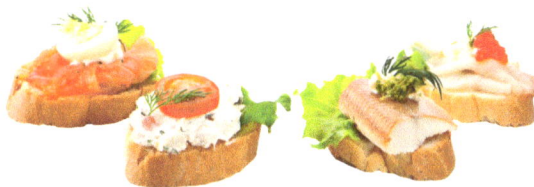

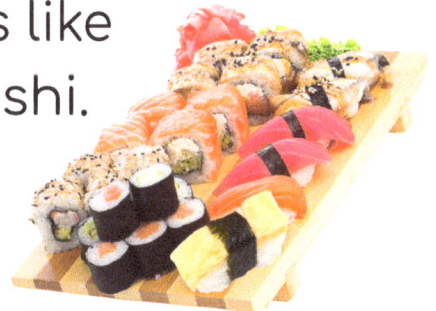

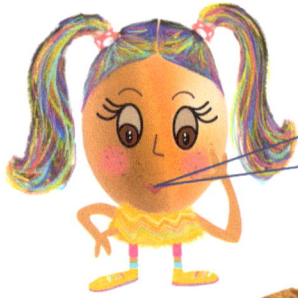

Aaaaand in...

pastries

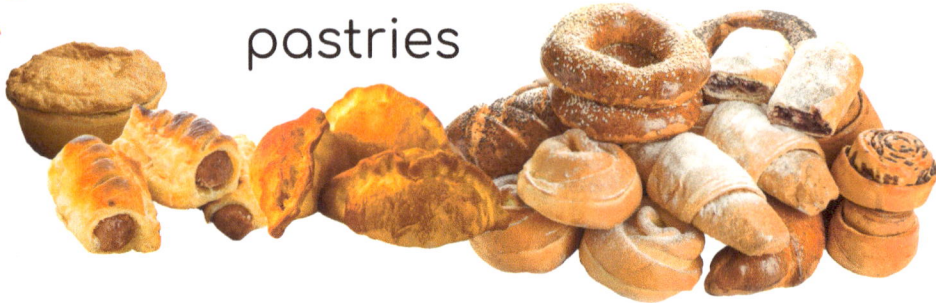

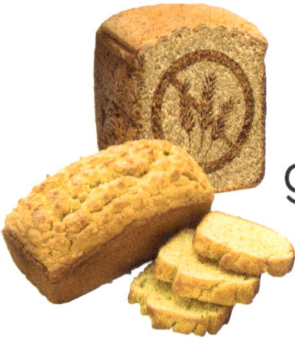

gluten free products

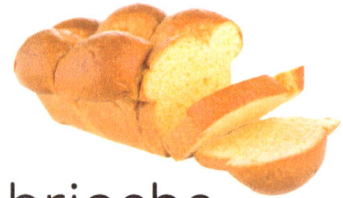

brioche

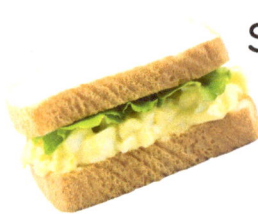

sandwiches, wraps and burgers

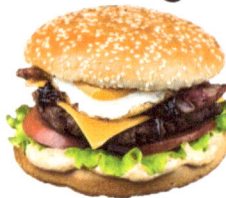

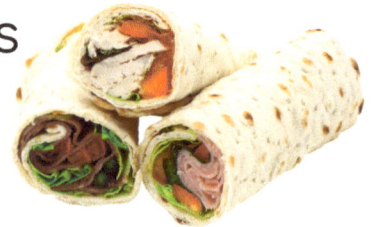

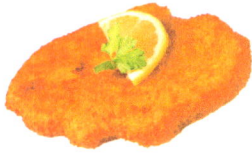 crumbed, stuffed and fried foods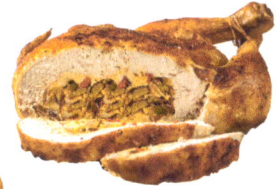

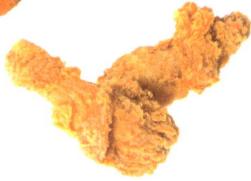 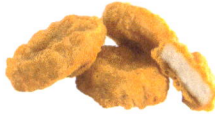 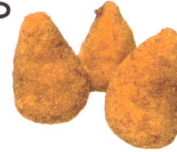

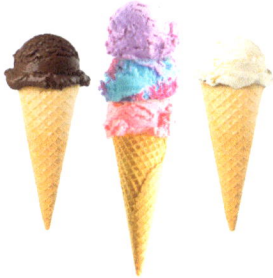 ice cream and gelato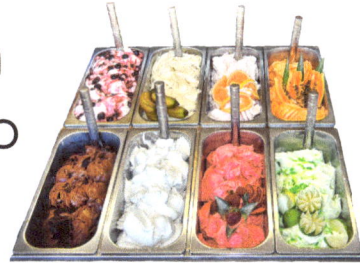

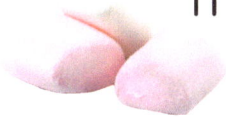 marshmallows

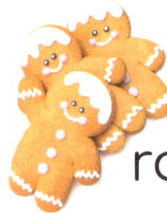 royal icing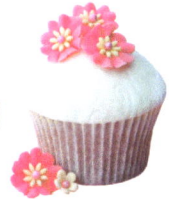

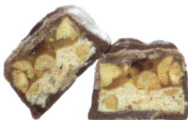 and nougat.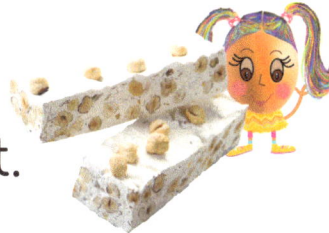

Peg - that's a lot of food you show up in!

Yeah. It is!

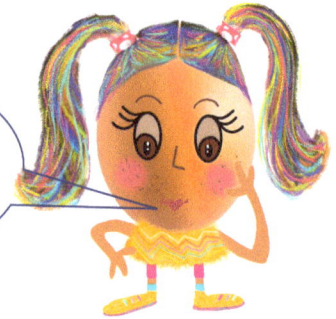

The good news is there are egg substitutes for baking or binding like

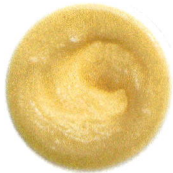

applesauce

buttermilk

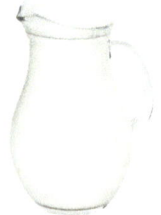

mashed banana

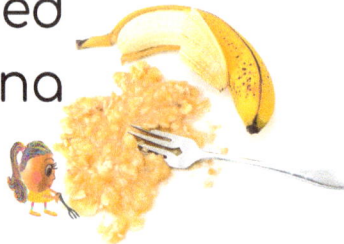

plain yogurt

aquafabba - liquid from a can of chickpeas

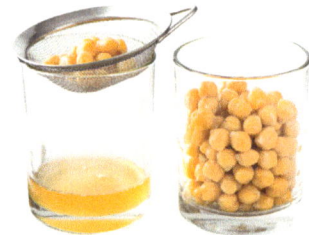

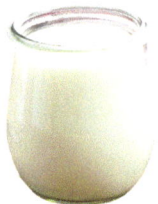

vinegar or lemon juice with baking powder

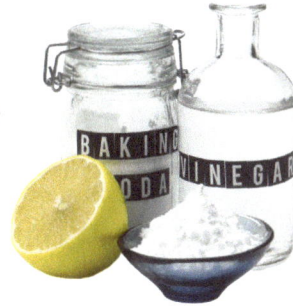

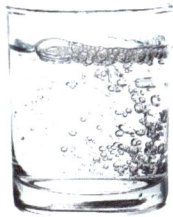

carbonated water

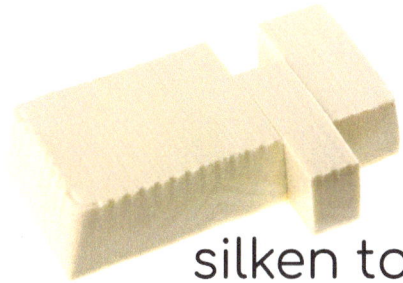

silken tofu

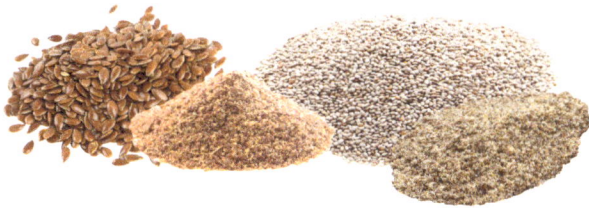

ground flaxseeds or chia seeds mixed with water

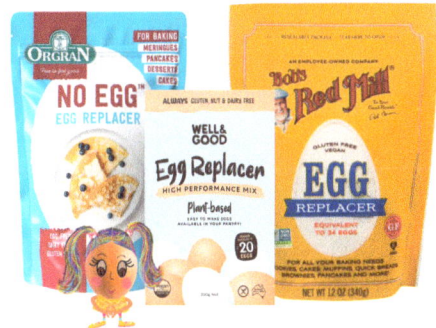

and commercial egg replacers.

Peg can leave traces in places like

food
factories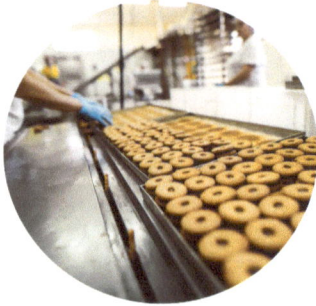

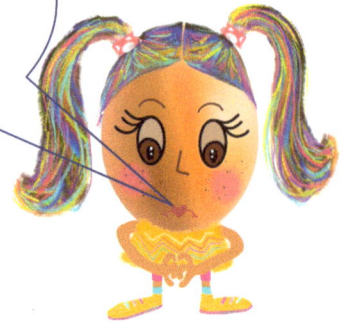

restaurants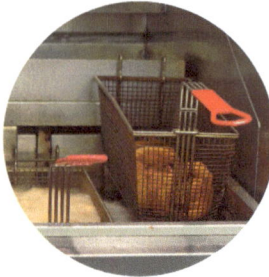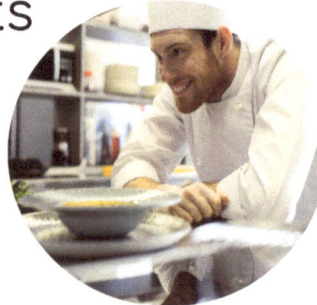

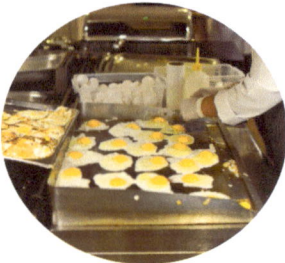

canteens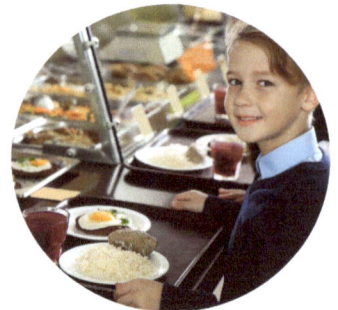

barbeques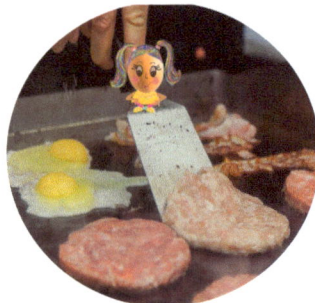

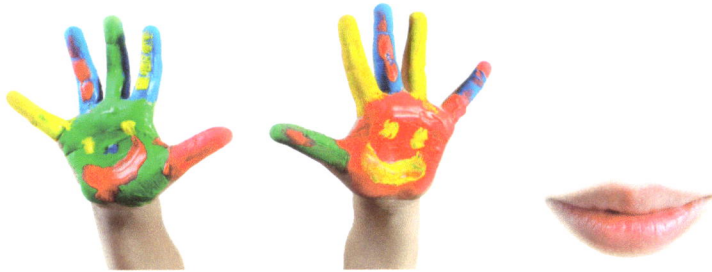

on hands and lips

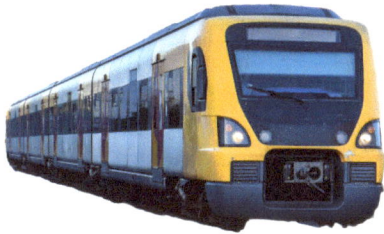

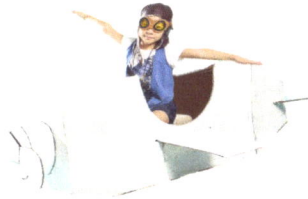

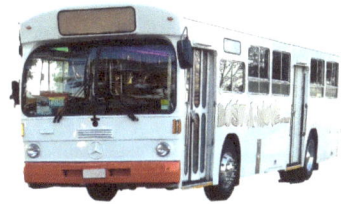

public transport

or at parties, play centres
and playgrounds.

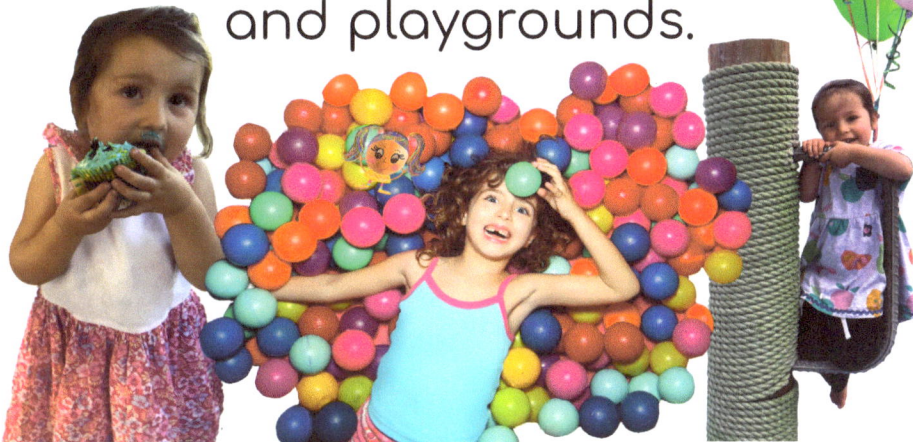

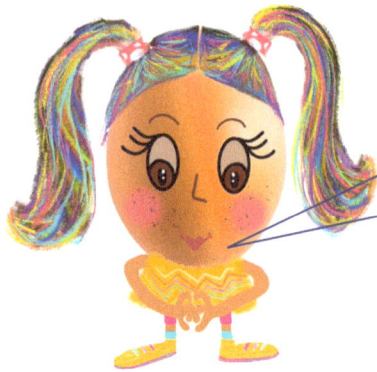

And, sometimes I can leave a trace on...

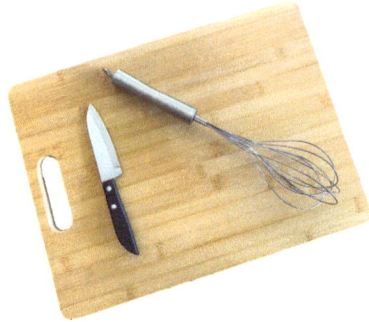

chopping boards

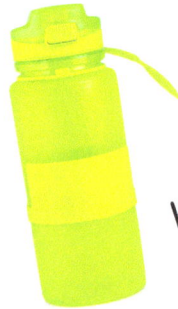

water bottles

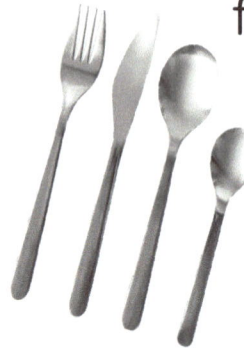

forks, knives, spoons

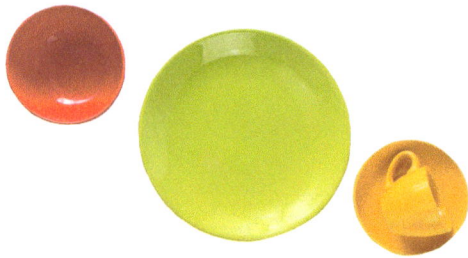

dishes, pots and pans.

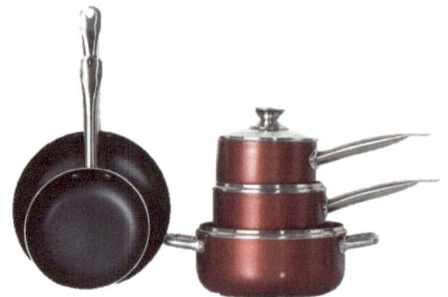

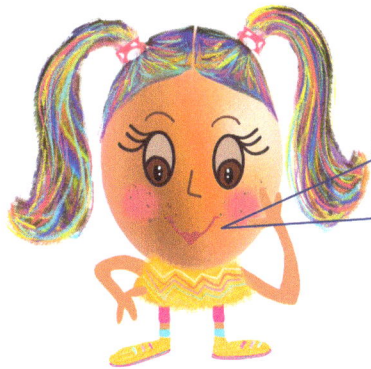

Or be an unexpected ingredient in ...

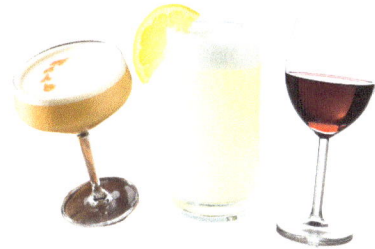

drinks

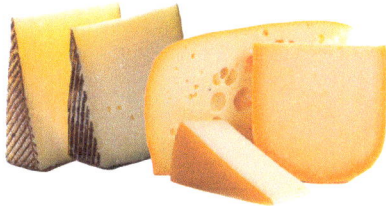

cheeses

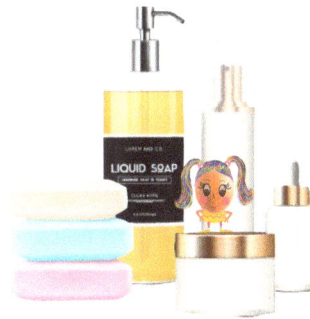

soaps and lotions

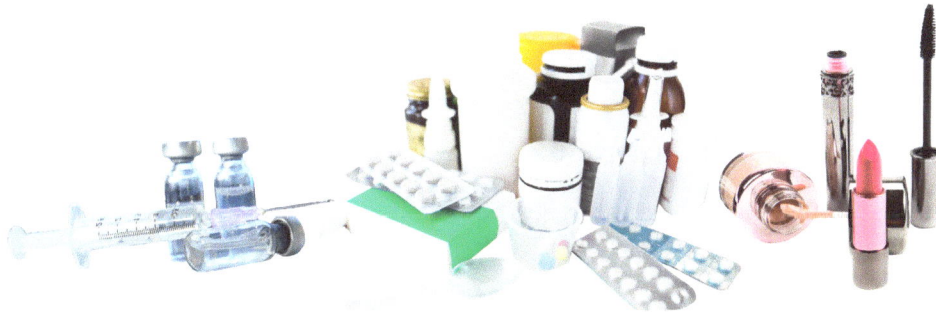

vaccines, medicine or makeup.

Albumen, Albumin, Apovitelin, Avidin, Flavoproteins, Globulin, Livetin, Lysozyme, Ovalbumin, Ovoglycoprotein, Ovomucoid/Ovomucin, Ovovitelin, Silici Albuminate or Simplesse are other ways "egg" may appear on a label.

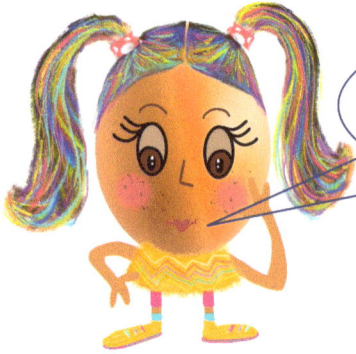

Egg allergies can be tricky...

That's right Peg.

Some people can be allergic to a teeny tiny trace of egg and avoid egg altogether.

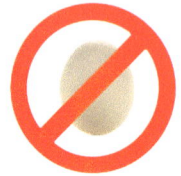

Others can safely eat eggs when baked in cakes or muffins

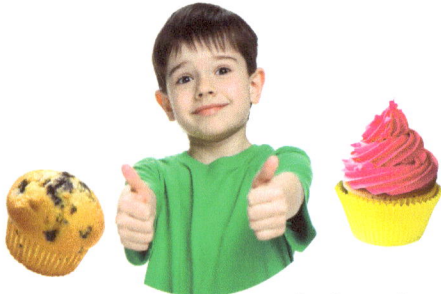

BUT NOT

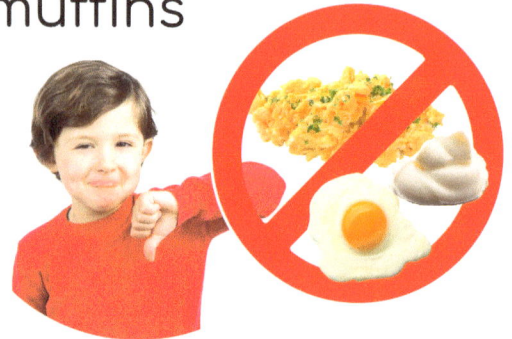

scrambled, fried or in mayonnaise!

Some people can safely eat
eggs laid by a duck
BUT NOT
eggs laid by a hen.

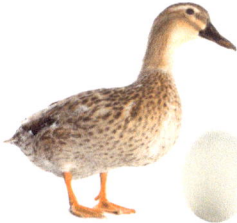

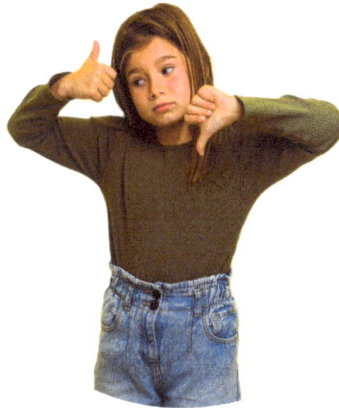

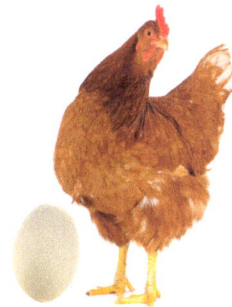

Every allergy journey is unique,
so it is important to know and share
how eggs affect **YOU**
and how **YOU** need to keep **YOURSELF** safe.

To keep everyone safe, whether they have allergies or not ...

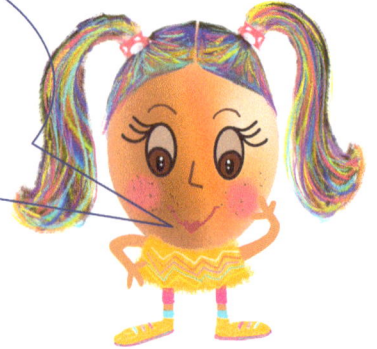

BEFORE

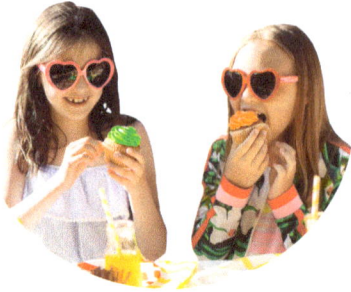

eating or sharing food

using drink bottles

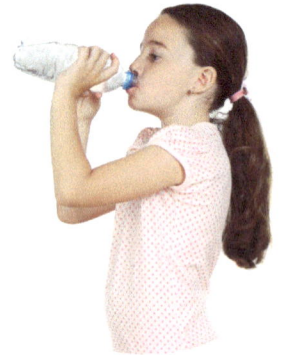

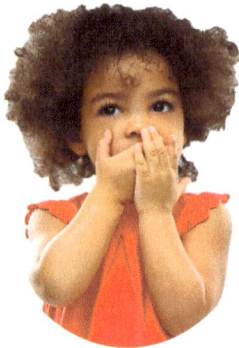

putting hands in or near mouths

or

kissing lips...

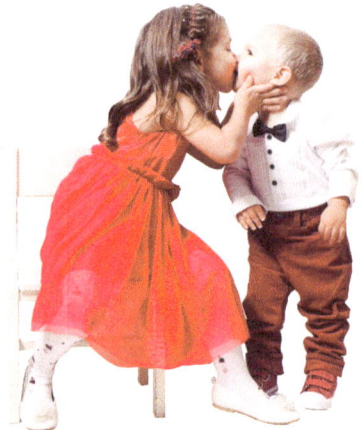

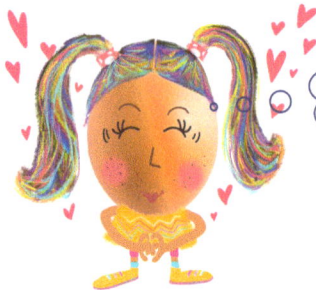

Naww-kissing!!

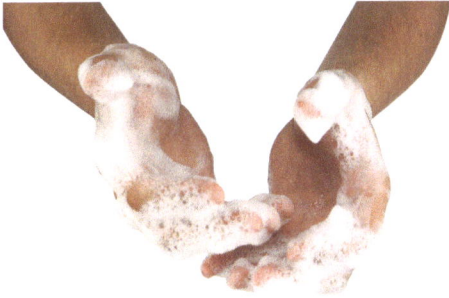

REMEMBER

Wash your hands, mouth, lips, dishes and surfaces.

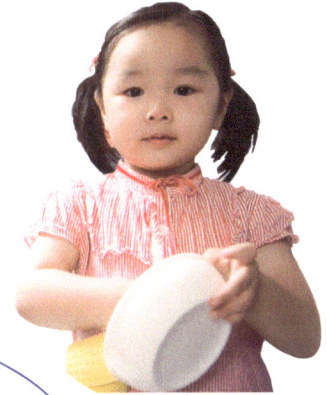

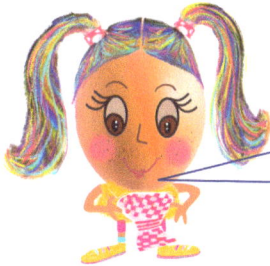

Soap and water works the best to remove allergen traces.

Read ingredient lists and allergy warnings on packaging when
1. buying
2. storing and
3. before using or eating!

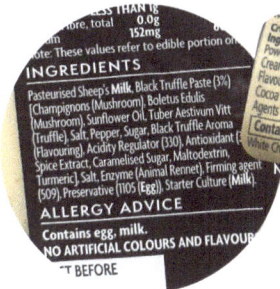

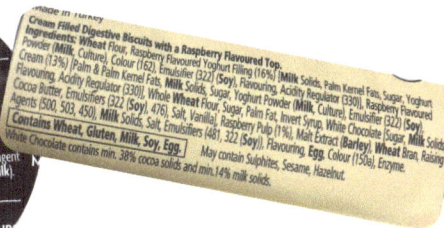

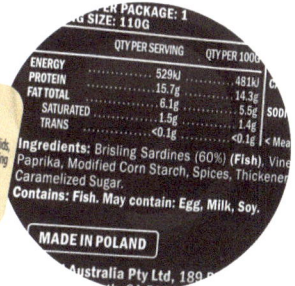

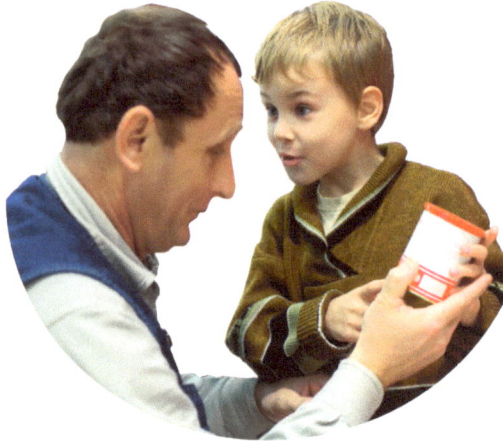

Talk to others about your allergies, risks and ways to keep you safe.

Let's see what can happen when someone allergic to Peg finds her by accident.

I can pop up in places unexpectedly sometimes...

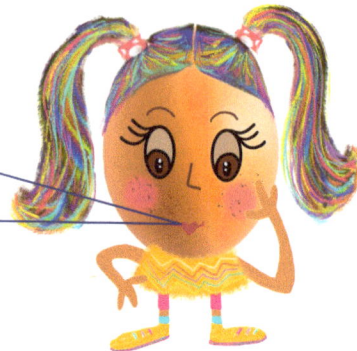

Peg can trigger unexpected reactions
for people with allergies, like

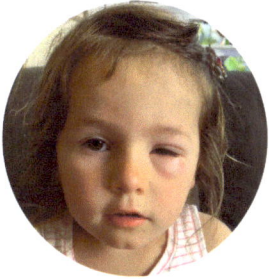 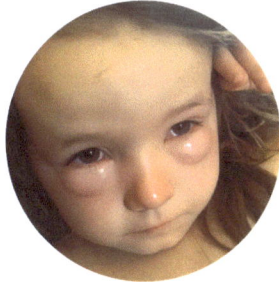 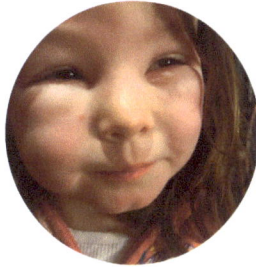

faces swelling
and puffing

itchy skin

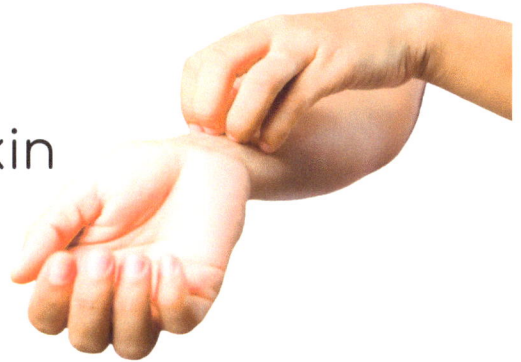

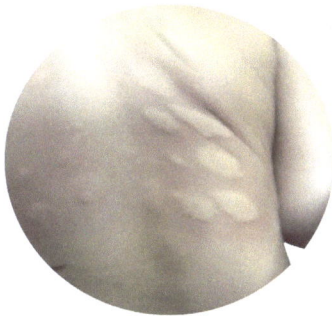

welts

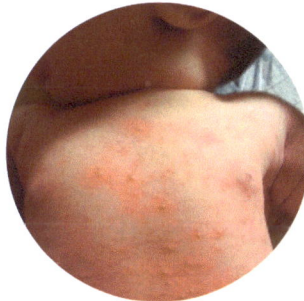

hives

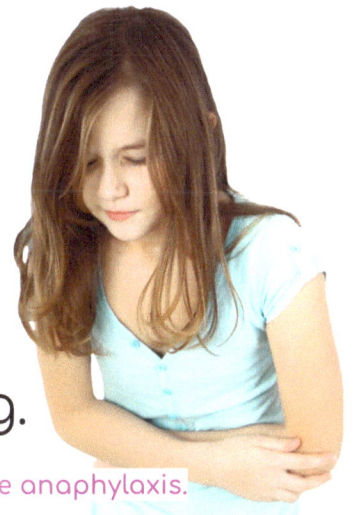

or vomiting.

Mild to moderate allergic reactions may not always appear before anaphylaxis.

Signs Peg may be causing
a severe allergic reaction are

trouble breathing

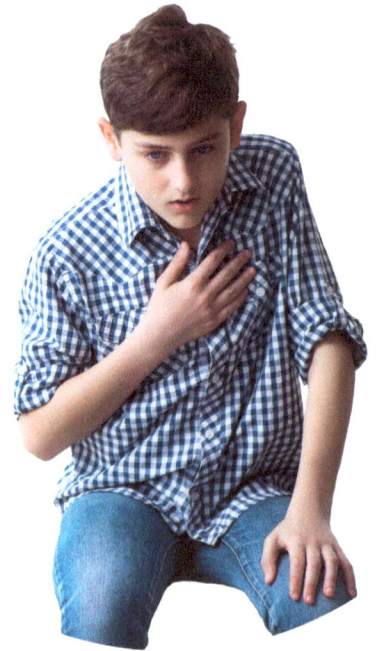

tight or tingly
throats

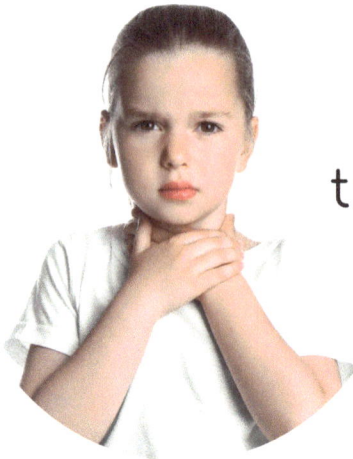

swelling tongues

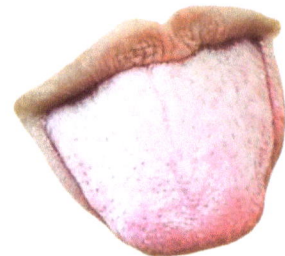

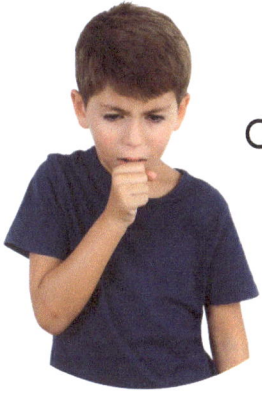

coughing or wheezing

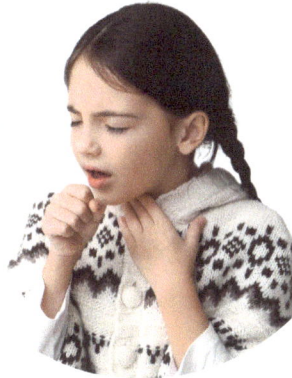

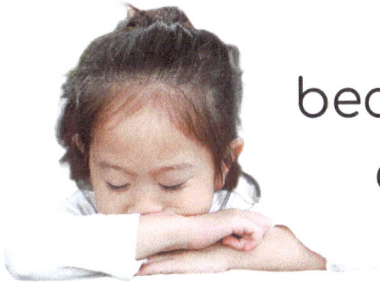

becoming pale or floppy

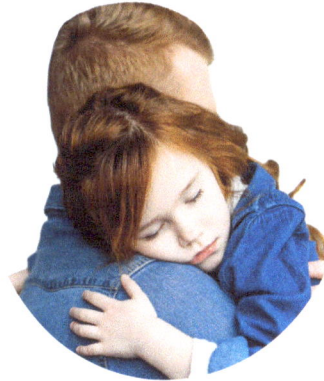

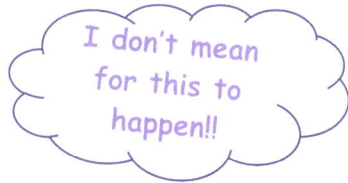

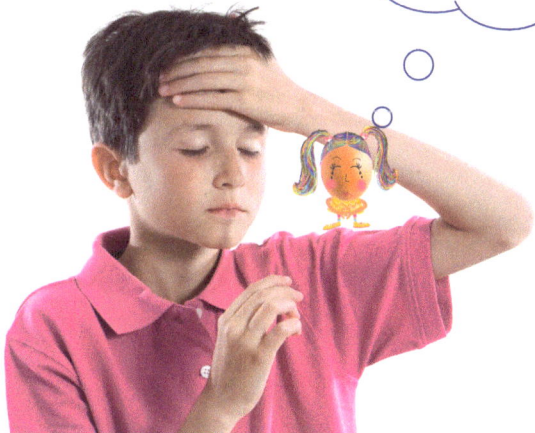

I don't mean for this to happen!!

feeling dizzy or collapsing.

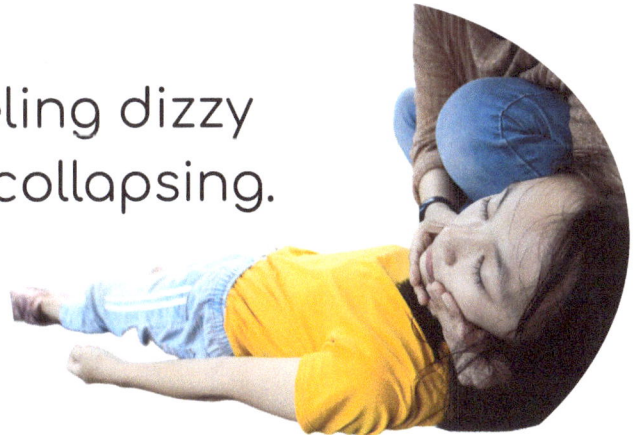

If you, a friend or a family member
have **ANY** of these reactions,
even for the first time,
tell an adult!

An adult is almost always around
but if not,
YOU can still help.

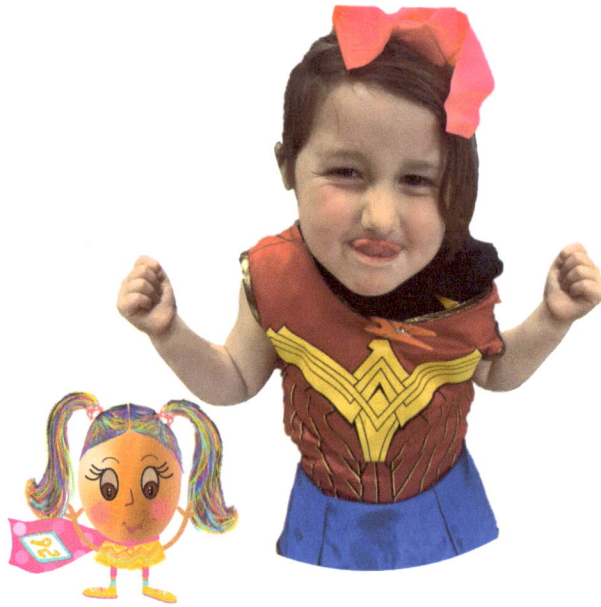

If a person is
having trouble breathing,
has swelling of the tongue,
tightness or tingling in the throat,
wheezing, is persistently coughing,
dizzy, pale, floppy or
has collapsed,
consider it to be
Anaphylaxis in action.

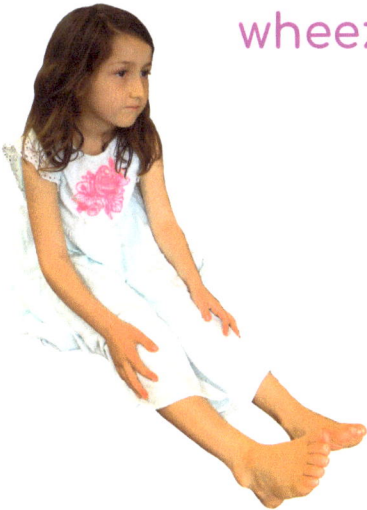

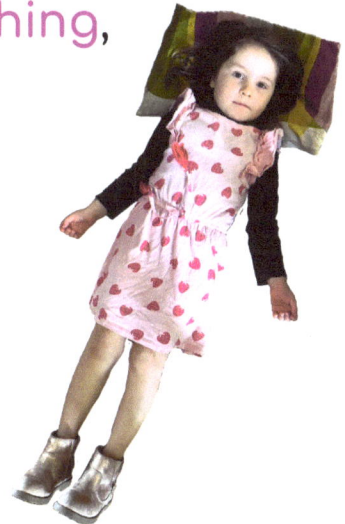

Make sure the person is
sitting or lying flat.

DO NOT let them stand or walk.

Remember anaphylaxis is life threatening!

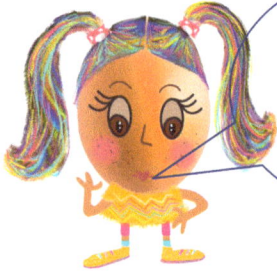

Action plans,
medications
and adrenaline pens
are kept at schools,
daycares,
in first aid kits
or carried by those
who have allergic and
anaphylactic reactions.

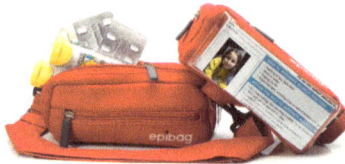

www.medibagaustralia.com

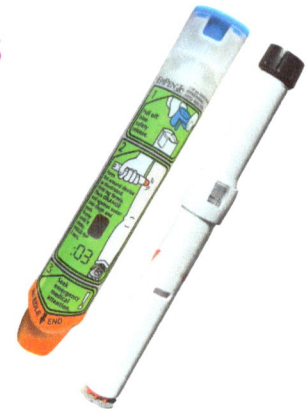

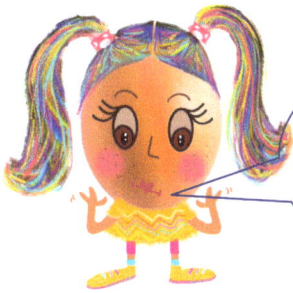

What's an Adrenaline Pen?

Epi-Pens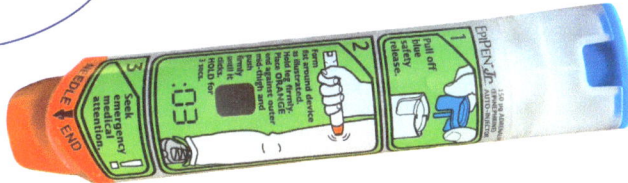

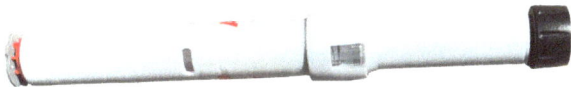 and Anapens

are two types of adrenaline pens that can be used during an anaphylactic reaction.

No Adrenaline Pen?

Stay calm

Make sure the person is sitting or lying flat

Monitor and call 000* for an ambulance

*000 (Australia) 111 (NZ), 112 (mobile/International Standard Emergency Number), 911 (US/CAN), 999 (UK)

If a person is also asthmatic - ensure the adrenaline pen is given FIRST, BEFORE administering asthma treatment. If in doubt, REMEMBER to follow their action plan if they have one and follow the emergency operator's instructions.

How to use an Epi-Pen

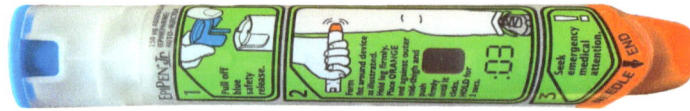

Grip the Epi-Pen
with one hand

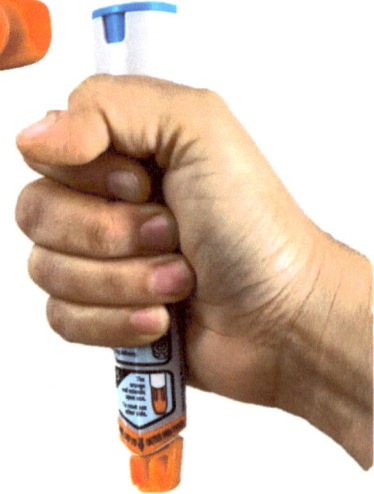

It's ok to use
through pants and jeans
just keep away
from pockets and seams

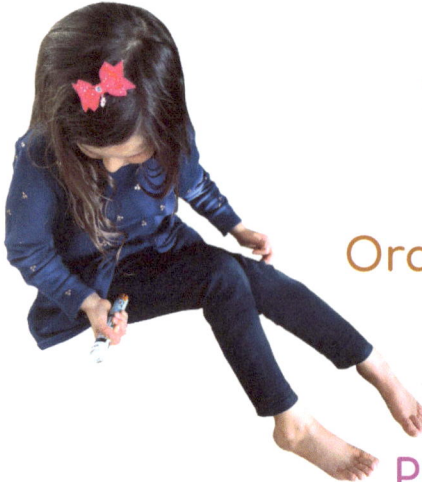

"**Blue** to the sky
Orange to the outer-mid-thigh"

Remove the **blue** cap

Push hard to hear the click
this **releases** the needle prick

Hold, and count 1 2 3
to set the adrenaline free

Remove the **Epi-Pen** gently

After administered, the orange end of the epi-pen will cover the needle prick.

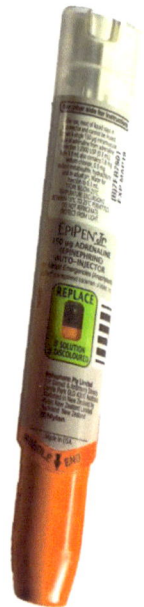

How to use an Anapen

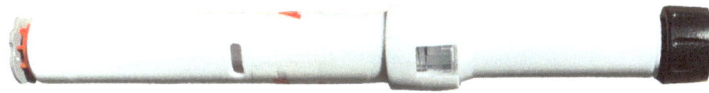

Pull off the **black** needle shield
and grey safety cap from the red button

It's ok to use
through pants and jeans
just keep away
from pockets and seams

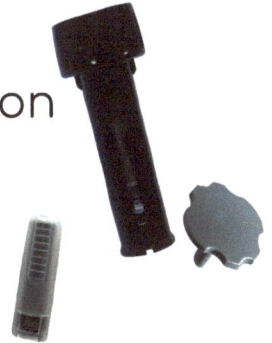

Place the needle end firmly
to the outer-mid-thigh

"White end on leg
press thumb on red"
to release the needle prick

Hold, and count 1 2 3
to set the adrenaline free

Remove the Anapen gently

Careful not to touch the exposed needle.
When possible, place the black needle shield over the needle.

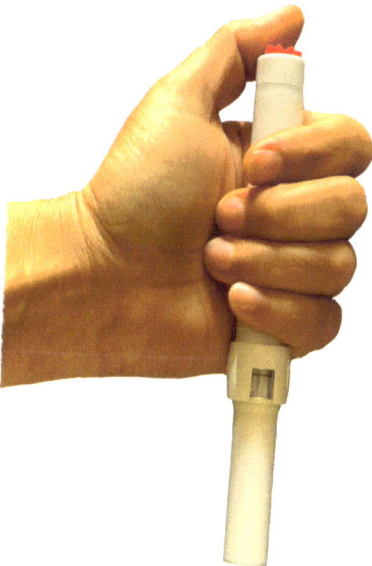

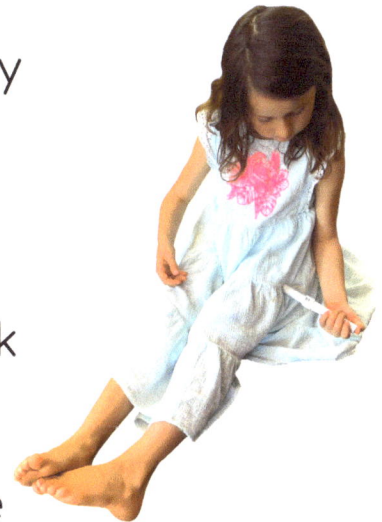

Don't leave the person alone

Use the phone to call 000*

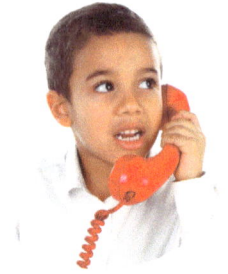

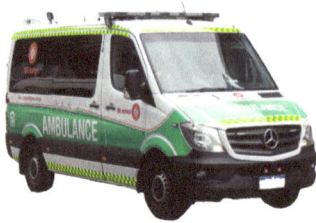

Ask for an ambulance
It's an emergency!

Follow the operator's instructions
until the ambulance arrives

While waiting,
a second adrenaline pen
can be used after 5 minutes
if signs don't improve

Then it's off to hospital
for monitoring
and more medical care

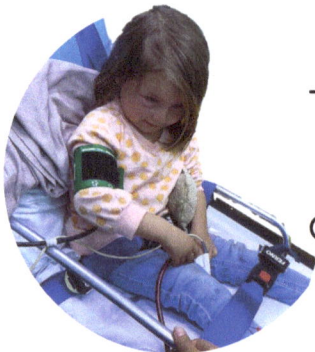

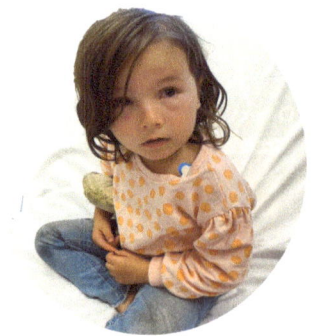

*000 (Australia) 111 (NZ), 112 (mobile/International Standard Emergency Number), 911 (US/CAN), 999 (UK)
Use CPR at <u>ANYTIME</u> if a person is unresponsive and not breathing normally.

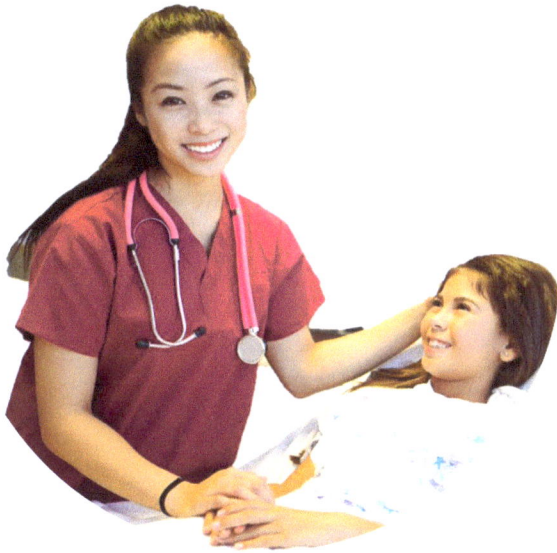

After hospital, finding out as much information about your allergens and how **YOU** react to them

will help **YOU** manage your allergies and keep **YOU** having fun.

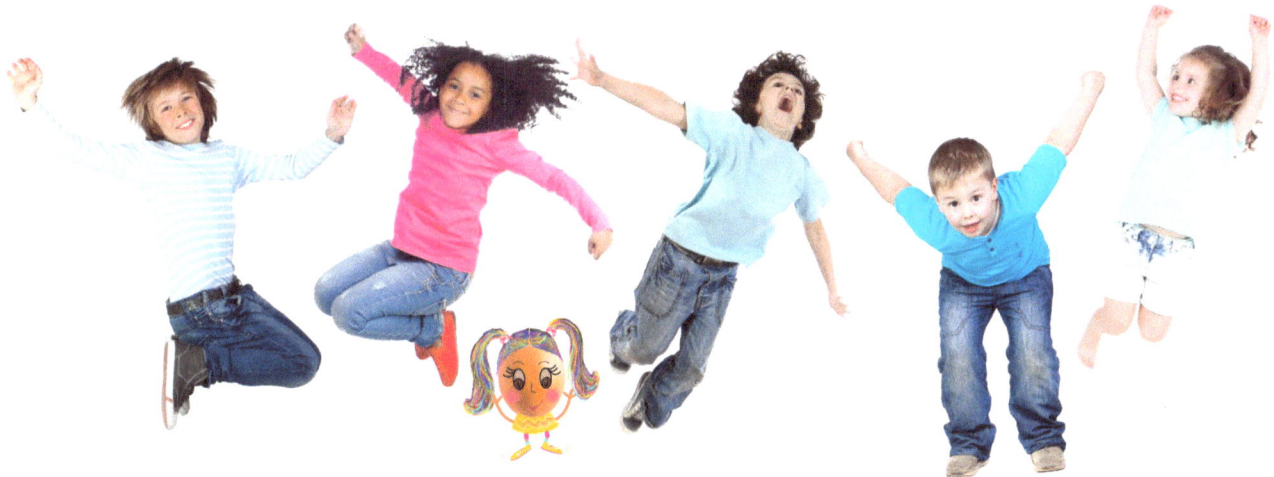

Allergists check for the likely cause of a reaction, assess risks and suggest treatments.

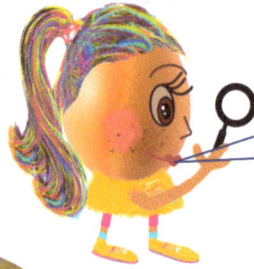

Allergists use tests like -

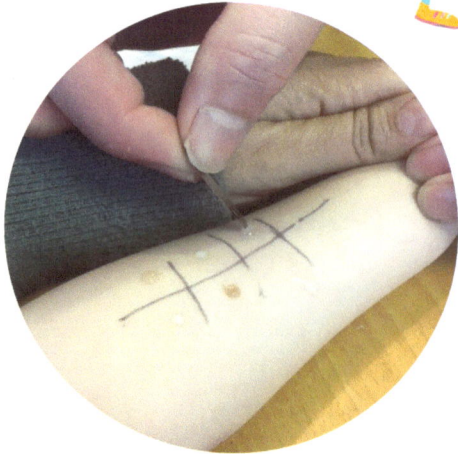

skin prick tests to measure reactions to drops of allergens

and blood tests to measure antibodies called IgE — short for *Immunoglobulin E.*

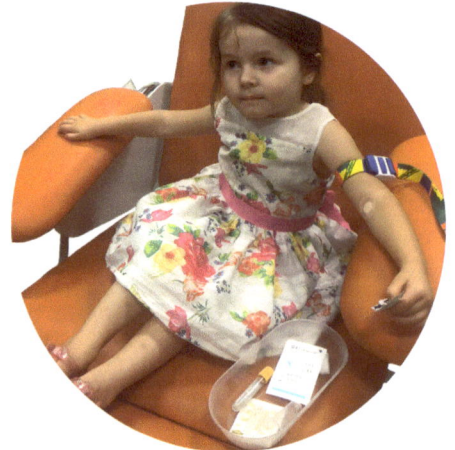

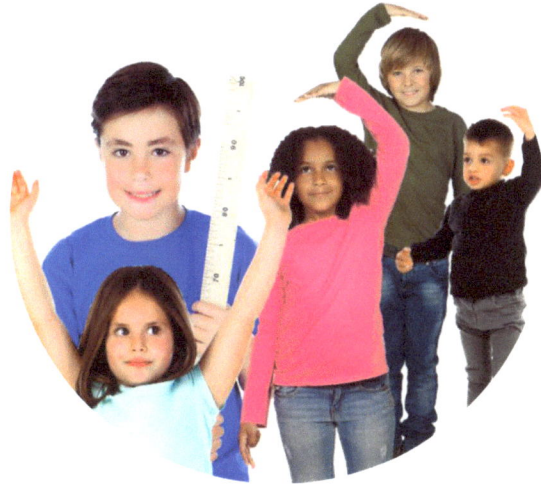

As bodies grow and change,
regular visits with allergists help to
safely test, tweak treatments

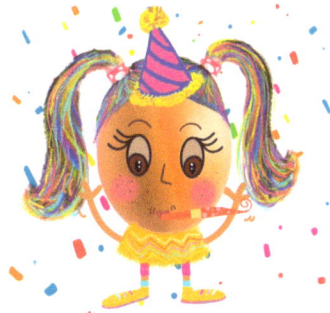

and may even show
an allergy
has been outgrown.

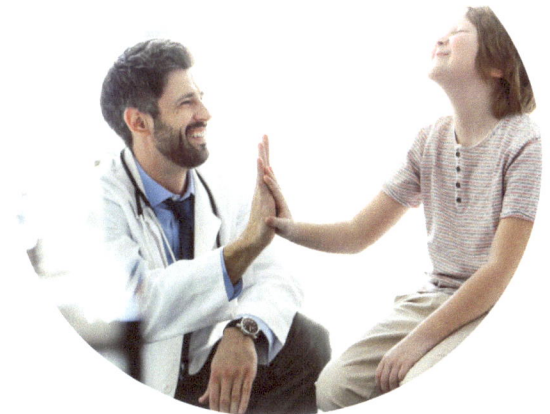

Extra Bits to Remember

If you're at risk of anaphylactic reactions have an adrenaline pen close by.

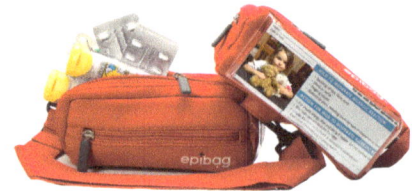

www.medibagaustralia.com

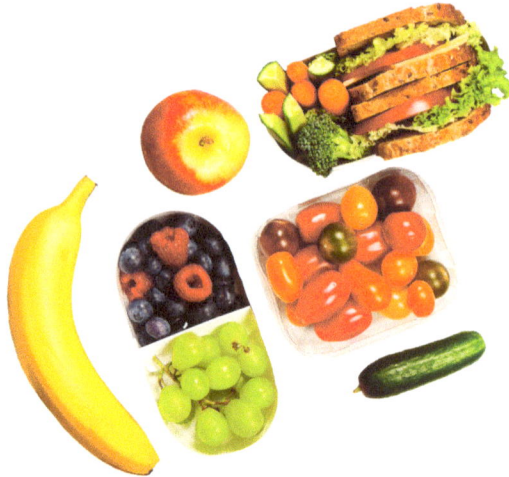

Pack your own safe food for when you are out and about.

If there isn't an adrenaline pen close by — *no food!*

Medicalert bracelets, bands and cards help inform and warn others.

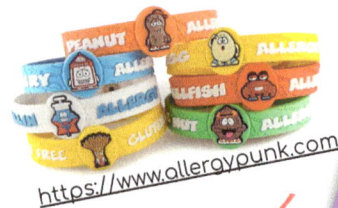

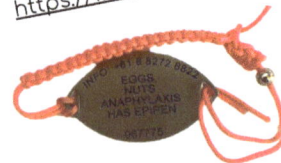

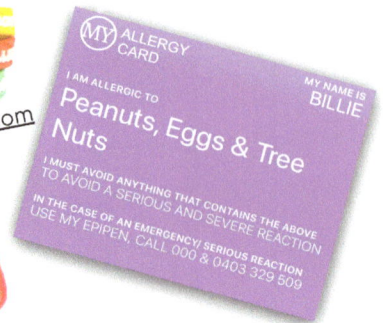

https://www.allergypunk.com

MY ALLERGY CARD

I AM ALLERGIC TO
Peanuts, Eggs & Tree Nuts

MY NAME IS
BILLIE

I MUST AVOID ANYTHING THAT CONTAINS THE ABOVE TO AVOID A SERIOUS AND SEVERE REACTION

IN THE CASE OF AN EMERGENCY/ SERIOUS REACTION
USE MY EPIPEN, CALL 000 & 0403 329 509

Make sure to tell people about the role eggs play in your day.

Ok Peg, time to say bye for now.

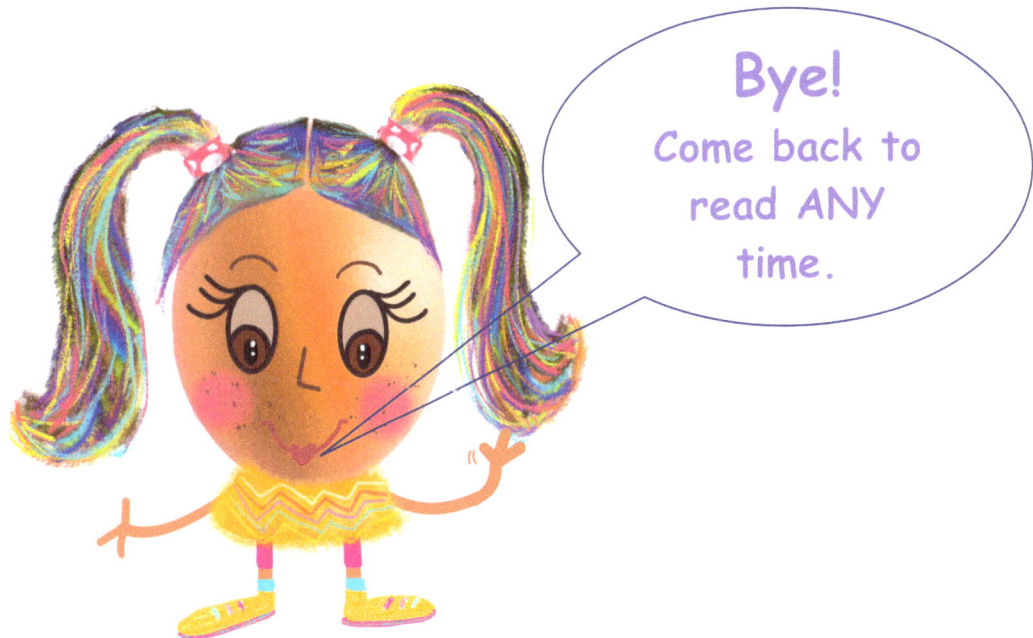

Bye!
Come back to read ANY time.

www.ingramcontent.com/pod-product-compliance
Lightning Source LLC
Chambersburg PA
CBHW041546260326

41914CB00016B/1566